# Strength Training For Seniors Over 60

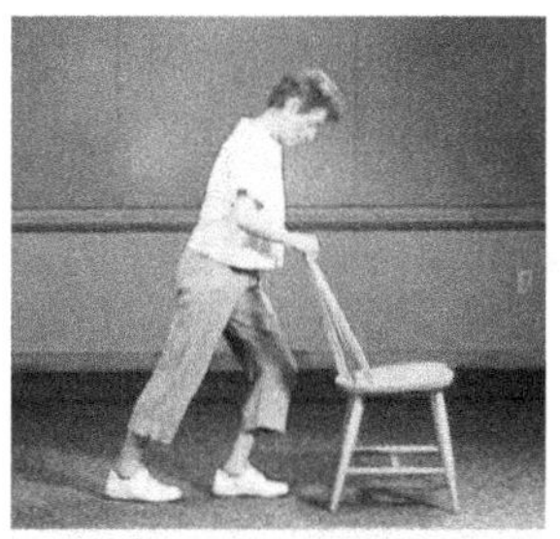

*Easy and Simple Home Workout to Improve Energy, Restore Balance and Retract the Effects of Aging.*

Written By

**Raymond V. Roberts**

# Table of Contents

# Introduction

The idea that growing older inevitably leads to weakness and deterioration has prevailed for far too long. However, this book dispels that idea. It reveals a route that demonstrates that getting older is just a number and that life may be just as colourful, active, and fulfilling in its second half. You'll go on a trip through the pages that follow that will enable you to realise your greatest potential and take advantage of the chance to succeed in your senior year of life.

The basic idea of our story is that growing older gracefully means becoming stronger and wiser rather than getting any weaker.

Strength training is a powerful tool that may help you stay young, improve your physical and mental health, and find vitality that you may have believed was gone forever.

This book is a thorough manual for seniors over 60 that is made to accommodate a range of fitness levels, from lifelong athletes to those who have never set foot in a gym. It provides you with a wealth of information, useful suggestions, and simple-to-follow exercises that can help you improve your general health, strength, and mobility.

In these pages, you will learn about the science underlying strength training, comprehend its numerous advantages, and find inspiration in the true-life stories of seniors who have overcome age-related challenges to welcome renewed energy. You will get the self-assurance and understanding necessary to start your own path to wellbeing and strength.

We'll go over the fundamentals of strength training, the value of diet, safe exercise methods, and injury prevention advice in the subsequent chapters. We'll present you a planned program that you can modify to fit your own requirements and skills. This book will walk you through every step of the process, whether your objective is to reclaim your independence, maintain an active lifestyle, or just enjoy the simple things in life.

Allow "Strength Training For Seniors Over 60" to serve as your pass to a self-determined future. You'll learn that growing older is no longer a barrier but rather an entrance to a life full of power, strength, and endless possibilities as we travel together. Being active becomes increasingly vital as you age. Frequent exercise can help you gain more muscle mass, manage pain or illness symptoms, maintain your independence, and lower your risk of developing neurological or cardiovascular problems.

**Would you like to discover the secret to a healthier, more active life. Unlock vitality and strength, no matter your age. Embrace the power of movement today!**

<u>CLICK HERE TO GET CHAIR PILATES FOR SENIORS</u>

# Chapter 1: Importance of Strength Training for Seniors.

Strength training is an essential part of general fitness for individuals of all ages, even seniors. Maintaining and even building physical strength becomes more crucial as we become older. We are going to examine the value of strength training for seniors, emphasising both its physical and psychological advantages.

**1. Preventing Muscle Loss:** Sarcopenia, or the progressive loss of muscle mass, is one of the most noticeable age-related changes. Seniors who engage in resistance activities, especially strength training, can counteract this muscle loss. Strength training increases total physical strength and functionality by providing a challenge to the muscles. It also promotes the development and repair of muscles.

**2. Improved Bone Health:** A significant concern among seniors is osteoporosis, a disorder that causes bones to weaken and fracture. Strength exercise increases the density and growth of bones, lowering the risk of fractures and preserving bone health. Exercises involving weight bearing, such deadlifts and squats, are especially useful for boosting bone density.

**3. Enhanced Stability and Balance:** Falls pose a serious risk to seniors and frequently result in injuries that have a substantial negative influence on their quality of life. Strength training lowers the risk of falls by enhancing stability and balance. This is accomplished by improving sense of balance and coordination and strengthening the muscles that support the joints.

**4. Improved Metabolism and Weight Management:** Strength training increases resting metabolic consumption of energy. Given that metabolisms tend to slow down in older adults, this can be quite helpful in controlling body weight and avoiding obesity. Reducing the risk of chronic diseases and maintaining a healthy weight are critical for general health.

**5. Better Joint Health:** By stabilising and protecting the joints, strong muscles help lower the risk of arthritis and joint problems. Strength training increases joint mobility and improves support for the surrounding structures, which helps reduce joint pain and discomfort.

**6.    Handling    Chronic    Conditions:** Diabetes, heart disease, and arthritis are just a few of the chronic illnesses that many seniors deal with. Strength exercise can lower blood pressure, improve insulin sensitivity, and relieve joint pain to help manage chronic disorders. To customise a strength training program to meet each person's unique health demands, it is imperative to consult with a healthcare professional.

**7. Improved Mental Health:** Research links physical exercise, particularly strength training, to better mental health. It can improve cognitive function, lower anxiety and depressive symptoms, and raise self-esteem. Seniors who engage in strength training can improve their overall quality of life by remaining physically active.

**8. Independence and Daily Activities:** To be independent in day-to-day activities, one must continue to be strong in muscles and able to function. Frequent strength training improves a senior's ability to carry out daily chores like grocery shopping, stair climbing, and getting in and out of chairs and beds.

**9. Social Engagement:** Since seniors frequently take part in group fitness courses or workouts with friends, strength training may be a social activity. In addition to promoting emotional health, social connection helps counteract feelings of isolation and loneliness.

**10. Longevity:** A number of researches have indicated that seniors who strength exercise might live longer. Maintaining strength and muscle mass is clearly linked to a better quality of life as one ages, even though the precise mechanisms are still unclear.

Strength exercise is essential to senior fitness. It has many advantages, including maintaining bone and muscle mass, enhancing metabolism, improving balance and stability, improving joint health, managing chronic illnesses, and having a favourable impact on mental health. Seniors who include strength training in their fitness routine can have improved independence and a higher quality of life, which will enable them to lead active and meaningful lives far into old age.

All organs and systems have a number of gradual, predictable, and progressive changes as we age. Throughout time, every person experiences physiological changes at the molecular, organ, and functional levels. Most organs reach their peak function in their third and fourth decades of life, after which there is a slow decline. Age-related symptoms are usually mild, unnoticed, and rarely interfere with day-to-day activities. However, homeostatic reserves decrease with ageing due to physiological changes. In times of increased demand or stress, usually brought on by disease, older individuals' reserves may not be sufficient to meet the demands of the particular circumstance. Over time, physiological changes are normal in most organs and should be differentiated from pathological changes brought on by illness. In the majority of cases, signs or symptoms point to an occult or visible illness in the elderly. Given how individualised and extremely diverse ageing is, biological and chronological ageing do not always match. The ideas of extraordinary longevity and maximum life span are explored. Physical activity and calorie restriction have long been linked to improved health and longer lifespans.

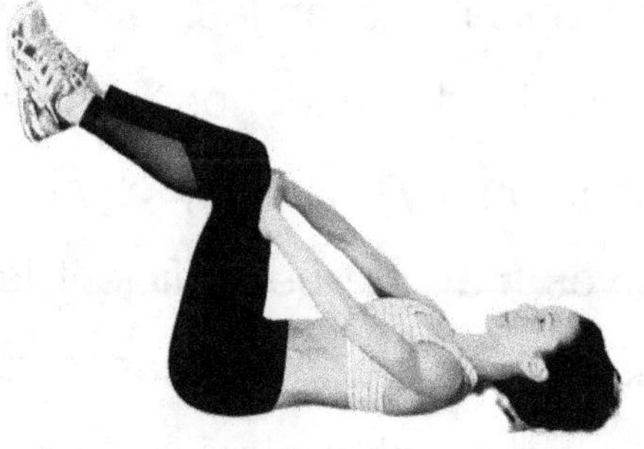

# 1.1.   Benefits of Strength Training for Seniors

For seniors, strength training provides a number of advantages, such as:

1.Enhanced Muscle Mass: Seniors who participate in strength training are able to preserve and grow their muscle mass, which is essential for overall functionality, mobility, and balance.

2.Better Bone Health: Strength training activities that involve weight bearing can increase bone density and lower the risk of osteoporosis and fractures.

3.Enhanced Metabolism: Strength training can increase muscle mass, which can help seniors manage diseases like diabetes and maintain a healthy weight.

4.Improved Joint Health: Pain and discomfort related to arthritis and other joint problems can be reduced by strengthening the muscles around joints.

5.Strength training has been shown to increase seniors' functional abilities, including their ability to move objects, climb stairs, and get out of a chair.

6.Improved Cognitive Health: Studies have shown that regular exercise, especially strength training, improves cognitive function and lowers the risk of diseases like dementia.

7.Enhanced Independence: Seniors' independence can be increased and their demand for daily life support can be decreased by maintaining their strength and mobility.

8.Enhanced Heart Health: When paired with cardiovascular activity, strength training can help lower blood pressure and enhance heart health.

9.Pain management: It can assist in reducing the chronic pain brought on by illnesses like arthritis or back pain.

Strength training can often result in an improved quality of life, enabling seniors to stay active and involved as they age.

# 1.2 Common Myths and Misconceptions about Strength Training for Seniors.

**Myth 1: I suffer from too many body aches and pains.**

Fact: Engaging in regular physical activity can help you effectively manage your body's aches and pains. It also strengthens you. Exercise not only increases strength but also counteracts the ageing-related loss of vitality. The key is to begin cautiously and slowly.

**Myth 2: I'm getting older, so it doesn't really matter if I exercise.**

Fact: Being active makes you feel and look younger and encourages independence. It also lowers the risk of getting a number of illnesses, including diabetes, high blood pressure, heart disease, stroke, Alzheimer's disease, and dementia.

**Myth 3: I find it really annoying. I'll never be as quick as I used to be.**

Fact: As you age, your body changes. Hormones, muscle mass, metabolism, and bone density may all fluctuate. Nevertheless, as you age, your power and performance level may unavoidably deteriorate. That doesn't mean that though, that you can't still gain from better health and the sense of achievement that comes from working out. It's recommended to start out slowly and adjust your workout regimen to your age-appropriate lifestyle goals. Never forget that there are more dangers to being inactive than benefits.

## Myth 4: Being active makes you more likely to fall.

In actuality, regular exercise can help increase muscular mass, boost endurance and strength, and stop the loss of bone mass. Your balance will consequently get better, lowering your chance of falling. Exercises for balance should be a part of any senior's fitness routine.

## Myth 5: Because I'm disabled I won't be able to exercise.

Fact: Engaging in physical activity presents specific difficulties for those with disabilities. Nonetheless, there are plenty of activities that are customised for them. To help with range of motion, muscle tone, flexibility, and cardiovascular health, they can lift weights, stretch, engage in chair aerobics, chair yoga, and chair Tai Chi. Wheelchair users may be able to participate in courses and other adaptive activities at many gyms or swimming pools.

**Myth 6: I'm past my prime.**

Fact: Exercise is something you should do at any age. It's never too late to start moving and enhance your general health. In actuality, compared to younger people, those who start exercising later in life get greater physical and psychological advantages. It's advisable to start with easy and gentle activities and work your way up if you've never tried exercising before or if it's been a while.Everyone should exercise.

# Chapter 2: Getting Started

Seniors who engage in strength training can experience significant improvements in their muscle mass, bone density, balance, and general quality of life. This is how to begin:

1.Speak with a Healthcare Professional: Make sure strength training is safe for you before starting any fitness program, especially if you have underlying medical concerns.

2.Establish Specific Objectives: Decide what you hope to accomplish with strength training. This could be greater bone health, higher muscle mass, or improved mobility. Setting clear objectives will help you stay motivated.

3.Select the Appropriate Workouts:
Pay attention to functional motions that enhance day-to-day tasks. Begin by performing bodyweight workouts such as push-ups, lunges, and squats. Add resistance training with dumbbells or resistance bands as you advance.

4.Acquire Correct Form: In order to avoid injuries, correct form is necessary. To ensure you are performing each exercise correctly, think about working with a certified fitness trainer.

5.Start Slowly: As you gain comfort and strength, progressively increase the intensity of your workouts by starting with modest weights and low resistance.

Be mindful of your body and avoid overdoing things.

6.Establish a Routine:

Consistency is important. Establish a regular exercise routine with the goal of doing strength training two or three days a week.

7.Warm Up and Cool Down: To avoid straining your muscles and increase flexibility, always warm up your muscles before exercising and cool down afterwards.

8.Balance and Flexibility: To increase stability and reduce the risk of falling, include exercises for both balance and flexibility in your regimen.

9.Track Your Progress: To keep track of your progress, keep a training notebook. This may inspire you and enable you to modify your regimen as necessary.

10.Nutrition and Hydration: To enhance your strength training efforts, have a well-balanced diet. Drink plenty of water and think about getting advice from a dietitian.

11.Rest and Recovery: In between sessions, give your muscles a chance to heal. Getting enough sleep is also essential for muscular growth and recuperation.

12.Safety first: Make sure the space where you exercise is secure and devoid of trip hazards. See your healthcare practitioner if you are in pain or uncomfortable.

## 2.1. Appropriate diet slows down the ageing process.

Although we cannot stop the clock, we may slow it down. Ageing is an inevitable aspect of life. Strength training, especially designed for seniors, along with a well-balanced diet is one of the most efficient strategies to achieve this. Our bodies naturally change as we age, leading to things like muscle loss, decreased bone density, and slowed metabolic rate. A reduction in general health and quality of life may result from these changes. On the other hand, elders can preserve their vitality and remain active for longer with a diet rich in particular nutrients and strength training.

## Diet's Contribution in Aging Gracefully:

1.Nutrient-Dense Foods: A senior's diet should prioritise foods high in nutrients. Fruits, vegetables, whole grains, lean proteins, dairy products, and dairy substitutes are some of these. Foods high in nutrients supply crucial vitamins and minerals that are needed for general health and well-being.

2.Antioxidants: These dietary components, which can be found in berries, nuts, and dark leafy greens, help fend off oxidative stress. This stress quickens the ageing process and aggravates cell damage.

Antioxidants can lessen the appearance of ageing by shielding cells from harm.

3.Drinking enough water is essential for keeping your skin looking good and your body functioning properly. Seniors who want to keep their skin smooth and improve their digestion should make a conscious effort to drink adequate water each day.

4.Protein: Maintaining muscle mass and strength need protein. Seniors who want to avoid the loss of muscle that commonly comes with ageing should make sure their diets contain enough protein.

5.Omega-3 Fatty Acids: These good fats, which are abundant in walnuts, flaxseeds, and fatty fish, contain anti-inflammatory and brain-healthy qualities that are essential for ageing gracefully.

# Chapter 3: Designing Your Strength Training Program

Once you have given it some thought, you are prepared to act on reasons for doing strength training and your objectives.

At this stage, you start getting ready for a fresh workout regimen.

You reserve the area needed in order to perform the workouts and purchase any tools you might require. You examine your plan to see how strength training might fit in and establish particular days and times for exercise.

Next stage is a thrilling time where you are picking up the exercises and performing them thrice a week. You're starting to make out the outcomes of your efforts. You observe physical modifications and notice that you feel more at ease and that your clothes fit a bit better, more robust, lively, and content. The action stage keeps on as long as you participate in the activity. However, after completing the exercises for roughly six months, you will have proceeded to the stage of maintenance.

Remaining On Path

At this point, strength training turns into a method of existence. By the time you get to this stage, chances are strong that It is difficult for you to contemplate skipping your workouts. As you find them entertaining and empowering, and you want to go on them because they give you a stronger, happier feeling. Shifting path self-sufficient and essential. You can discover that you're engaging in activities you had given up on years earlier, including golf and gardening, canoeing, dancing etc. As you advance, you might additionally incorporate fresh strengthening routines and new pursuits in your life.

If you want to transform your life in a way that will make sense, It's beneficial to take some time to consider what inspires you. Why do you wish to engage in strength training?

What are your individual objectives? What challenges could prevent you  and how could you get past them? It's a smart idea as well to picture yourself succeeding and think about how you might honour your accomplishments.

The different types of Strength Training Exercises For Seniors are:

1.Bodyweight Exercises: These exercises, which include push-ups, planks, squats, and lunges, use your own body weight as resistance. They enhance stability and balance.

2.Resistance Bands: Perfect for elders, these elastic bands offer resistance during workouts. Leg lifts, rows, and bicep curls are a few possible exercises.

3.Movements with Light Dumbbells: You can perform movements like bent-over rows, tricep extensions, and seated overhead presses with light dumbbells.

4.Machine-Based Workouts: in order to target specific muscle areas while maintaining stability, seniors can safely use resistance machines at a gym.

5.Functional Movements: To increase functional strength, perform exercises that replicate commonplace tasks like carrying groceries or getting out of a chair.

6.Exercises that are isometric—such as wall sits or planking—involve retaining a position and can increase strength and stability without putting undue strain on the joints.

7.Tai Chi: This low-impact martial technique improves muscular endurance, flexibility, and balance.

8.Yoga: The stretches and positions in yoga improve flexibility and tone muscles with light effort.

9.Water Aerobics: The buoyancy of the water provides resistance for strength training while lessening joint stress.

10.Exercises with Elastic Bands: Leg lifts, seated rows, and other strength-training exercises can be performed using elastic bands.

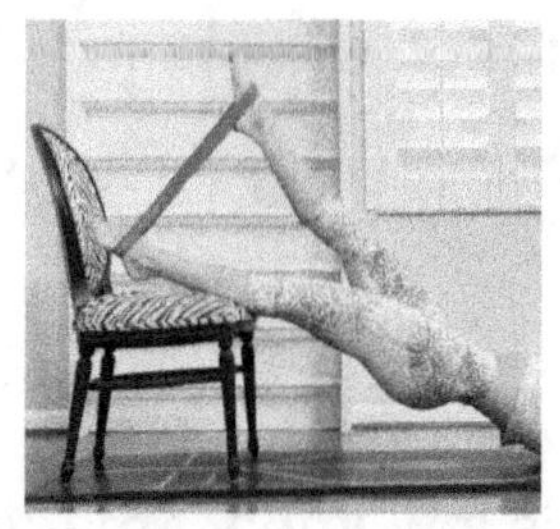

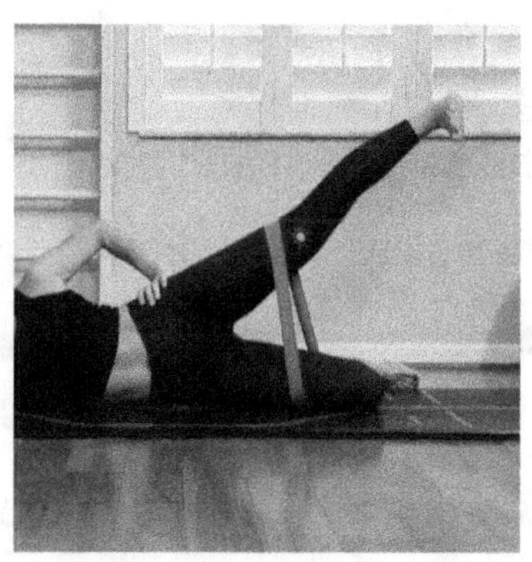

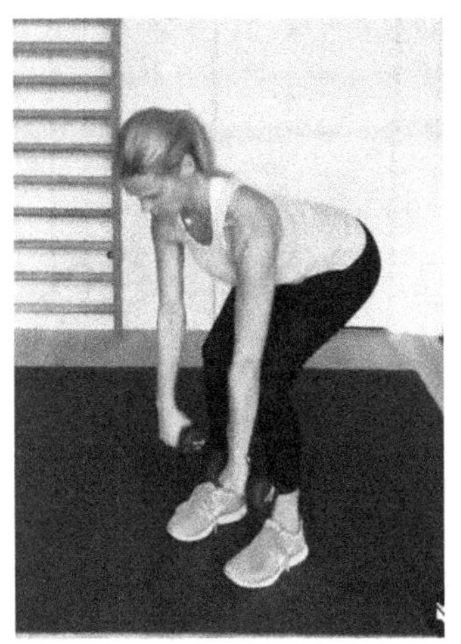

# 3.1 Warm-Up and Cool-Down Routines

**Warm-up Routine:**

- Light Aerobic Activity: To raise heart rate and blood flow, start with five to ten minutes of low-impact aerobic activity, such as walking or stationary cycling.
- Joint Mobility Exercises: To increase range of motion and lower the chance of injury, gently rotate and stretch your joints.
- Bodyweight Exercises: To work the primary muscle groups, incorporate bodyweight exercises like arm circles or air squats.

- Dynamic Stretches: To better prepare the muscles for action, incorporate stretches like arm circles and leg swings.
- Gradual Intensity: Start with smaller weights or resistance bands and gradually raise the intensity of your workouts.

**Seniors' Cool-Down Routine:**
- Stretching Static: Hold each major muscle group stretch for a duration of 15 to 30 seconds.
- Deep Breathing: To ease muscle tension and promote relaxation, engage in deep breathing exercises.
- Gentle Self-Massage: To ease any tension or stiffness in your muscles, practice self-massage techniques.

- Hydration is important for muscle recovery, so drink plenty of water to stay hydrated.
- Take some time to think back on your workout and unwind mentally and physically.

# Chapter 4: Targeting Specific Muscle Groups

## 4.1 Upper Body Exercises

1. Chaired Dumbbell Lift:

   - With your feet flat on the floor and your back straight, take a seat in a strong chair.
   - With your hands pointing forward, hold a dumbbell at shoulder height in each hand.
   - Raise the dumbbells until your arms reach their maximum length.
   - Reposition the weights so they are shoulder height.

- Perform 10–12 repetitions in two or three sets.

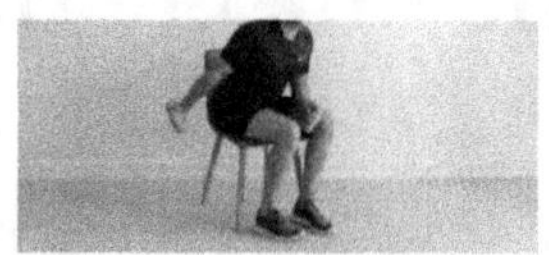

*Chair Dumb bell lift.*

2. Bicep Curls:

- With your back straight and your arms by your sides, grip a dumbbell in each hand while you sit or stand.
- Curl the weights slowly toward your shoulders while maintaining your hands facing forward.
- Reposition the weights so that your arms are fully extended.
- Perform 10–12 repetitions in two or three sets.

3.Lateral Raising:

- With your back straight and a dumbbell at either side, take a seat in a chair.
- Bend your elbows slightly and raise your arms to shoulder height.
- Relative to your sides, lower your arms.
- Perform 10–12 repetitions in two or three sets.

4.Rows :

- Stretch your legs wide, sit on a chair or bench, position a resistance band under your feet, and grip the ends of the band.

- Apply pressure to your shoulder blades by pulling the band in the direction of your waist.
- Release the band gradually.
- Perform 10–12 repetitions in two or three sets.

5. Chest Press Exercise:

- With a dumbbell at chest height in each hand, place yourself on a mat or bench and lie on your back.
- Raise the weights until your arms reach their maximum length.
- Reposition the weights so they are chest height.
- Perform 10–12 repetitions in two or three sets.

6. Wall Push-Ups

- With your arms at shoulder height and your palms flat on the wall, take a stance facing the wall.

- Push yourself back to the beginning position after bending your body toward the wall.

- Perform 10–12 repetitions in two or three sets.

7 Prone Y Raises:

- Arms extended above in a "Y" configuration, lie face down on a mat. (You can also do this exercise while standing and spice it up with a resistance band as shown below.)

- Keeping your shoulder blades together, raise your arms off the floor.

- Return your arms to the floor.

- Perform 10–12 repetitions in two or three sets.

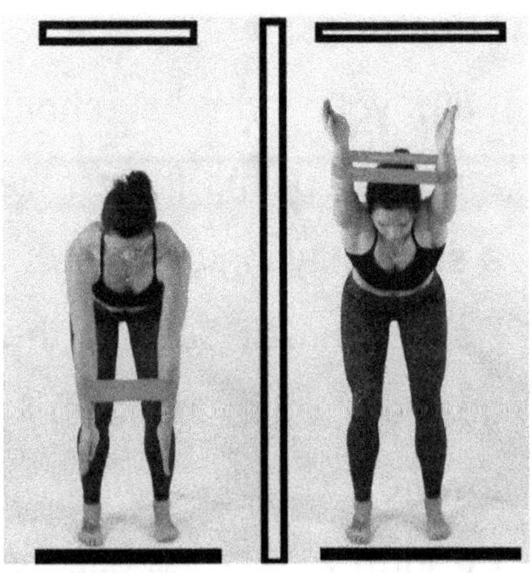

8. Extending the Tricep:

- With both hands held overhead, hold a dumbbell while sitting upright in a chair.

- To reduce the weight behind your head, bend your elbows.

- Reach out and lift the weight back up.

- Perform 10–12 repetitions in two or three sets.

To avoid injury, always pay attention to proper form and begin with lower weights or resistance. You can progressively raise the weight or resistance and the number of sets and repetitions as your strength and confidence grow.

## 4.2 Lower Body Exercises

1.Weightlifting Squats:

- Place your feet hip-width apart as you stand.
- Assume that you are going to sit down and gradually lower your body.
- Rise once more. Be careful not to bend your knees too much forward.

2.Wall Seating:

- Put your back to a wall while standing.
- Slide along the wall at a slow pace until your knees form a straight angle.
- As long as you can, maintain this posture, then get back up.

3.Leg Lifts:

- For balance, cling to a wall or chair.
- Lift one straight leg and bring it to the side or back.
- Retrace your leg's descent.

4. Step ups:

- Locate a solid bench or step.
- With one leg, step up onto it and then step back down.
- Continue with the opposite leg.

5. Lunges

- Step forward, or step backward.
- A correct right angle should be formed by your knees.
- Take care not to bring your front knee too far forward.
- Return to where you were standing before.

6.Calf Raises:

- Place your feet hip-width apart as you stand.
- Raising your heels as high as you can will help.
- Reposition your heels lower.

7.Chair Squats:

- Perch on a supportive chair.
- Using your leg muscles, get yourself out of the chair.
- Resuming your seat, then repeat.

## 4.3    Core      Strengthening Exercises

1.Seated Leg Lifts:

- With your back erect, take a seat in a firm chair.
- Stretch out one leg and raise it off the ground.
- Hold it for a short while before lowering it.
- Continue with the opposite leg.
- Repeat steps 10–15 for each leg.

2.Seated Marches:

- With your feet flat on the ground and your back straight, take a seat in a chair.

- Raise one knee to a comfortable level, then bring it back down.
- Continue with the opposite knee.
- Perform 15–20 knee lifts in succession.

3.Bridge Exercise:

- Lying on your back, place your feet flat on the floor and bend your knees.
- Raise your hips off the floor so that your shoulders and knees are in a straight line.
- After a little period of holding, drop your hips.
- Do between 10 and 15 reps.

4.Plank on the Wall:

- With your hands flat on the wall and your arms shoulder-width apart, take a stance facing a wall.

- Take a step back so that your head and heels form a diagonal line.
- Hold this position for twenty to thirty seconds.
- As your strength increases, gradually extend the duration.

5.Chair Twists:

- With your feet flat on the ground and your knees bent, take a seat on a chair's edge.
- For stability, grip the chair's sides.
- Turn your upper body slowly to one side, then back to the centre.
- Continue on the opposite side.
- Twist on each side ten to fifteen times.

**More Exercises:**

1. Toe Stand.

The toe stand exercise is for you if going for a stroll in the park doesn't seem easy or fun anymore! By strengthening your calves and ankles and regaining stability and balance, it will contribute to making your park stroll enjoyable and stress-free.

- Approach a solid chair or counter with your feet shoulder-width apart. For balance, use the counter or chair.
- As you count to four, slowly push up as far as you can onto the balls of your feet. For two to four seconds, maintain this stance.
- Next, as you count to 4, gently return your heels to the floor.
- For one set, repeat ten toe stands. For roughly a minute, rest. Finish a

second set of ten toe stands after that.

- Make sure you do not lean on the counter or chair, use the chair for balance only.
- Breathe consistently while performing the activity.

2.Marching Fingers.

You will be using your fingers, hands, and arms to walk during this exercise. This will improve your grip and upper body strength. It will also improve the range of motion in your shoulders, back, and arms.

Place your feet on the floor and either stand or sit forward on a chair.
Place your feet shoulder-width apart.

**Movement 1:** Picture yourself standing in front of a wall. Ascend the wall slowly with your fingers until your arms are above your head. Wiggle your fingers while keeping your arms raised for approximately ten seconds. Then, carefully walk them back down.

**Move 2:** Afterwards, make an effort to touch your hands behind your back. Try to get as close as you can to the opposing elbow with each hand, if at all possible. You should feel a stretch in your arms, chest, and back after holding the pose for ten or so seconds. Release your arms.

3. Improved Grip Strength.
Having arthritis can make it difficult for you to hold onto objects or pick them up. You might also wish to incorporate a grip workout if your grip strength is a concern in

order to strengthen and loosen up your hands. The majority of individuals already have the equipment at home, and the exercise is easy to perform while reading or watching TV.

Tennis ball, racquetball, or "stress" ball as equipment.

Time: Under five minutes.

Exercise: While seated or standing, hold a ball with one hand and squeeze it as firmly as you can, slowly, and hold the squeeze for three to five seconds. Release the squeeze gradually.
After a brief break, perform the exercise ten times. Perform two sets of ten squeezes with the other hand after switching hands.

Depending on how your hands feel, you can perform this exercise daily or every other day. You might wish to skip a day if they are sore or stiff.

4.Above-the-head press

This beneficial workout works a number of shoulder, upper back, and arm muscles. Additionally, it can assist strengthen the backs of your upper arms and facilitate reaching up into high cabinets for goods.

- Place your feet shoulder-width apart whether standing or sitting. Take up a dumbbell with one hand. Raise your hands until the dumbbells are parallel to the floor and level with your shoulders, keeping your forearms and palms facing forward.

- As you count to two, slowly raise the dumbbells over your head until your arms are completely extended. Take care not to bend your elbows.

- Hold on. Then, as you count to four, carefully lower the dumbbells back to shoulder level while bringing your elbows close to your sides.

- For one set, repeat ten times. For roughly a minute, rest. After that, finish a second set of ten repetitions.

**Ensure that:**

You don't flex your wrists.
Let your shoulders and neck drop.
Maintain a small bend in your arms instead of locking your elbows.

Keep the dumbbells from moving too far in front or behind your body.

Breathe consistently while performing the activity.

5.Sided Hip Raise:

Your hip, thigh, and buttock muscles are the focus of the side hip raise. This workout strengthens and tones your hips, which are more prone to breaking as you get older. It also tightens and moulds your lower body.

- Place your feet slightly apart and point your toes forward while standing behind a sturdy chair. Don't lock your knees, but maintain a straight leg posture.
- While you count to two, slowly raise your left leg out to the side. Maintain

a straight leg, but remember not to lock your knee.

- Hold on. Then, as you count to four, carefully return your left foot to the ground.
- For one set, repeat 10 times with the left leg and 10 times with the right. For roughly a minute, rest. After that, perform ten more reps of each leg in a second set.

6.Back, Neck, and Shoulder Stretches.

The neck, back, and shoulders are a further group of muscles that are prone to tension and stress. This gentle stretch targets these muscles.

Stretch before and after strength training, as well as whenever you do an activity that causes stiffness, like working at a desk. You'll discover that it will energise you.

1. Place your hands in front of you, stand (or sit) with your feet shoulder-width apart, and your knees straight but not locked. Turn your hands so that the palms are facing downhill. After that, elevate your arms to a level with your chest.

2. Feel a stretch in your upper back, shoulders, and neck as you press your palms out from your body.

3. Maintain the stretch while breathing deeply for a leisurely 20 to 30 seconds.

Repeat after releasing the stretch.

By the time you can perform the exercises in this book, you will probably have increased your strength and muscle mass and enhanced your flexibility, balance, and coordination.

Congratulations, getting started and maintaining a strength-training program is a huge accomplishment. If you want to reap the many advantages of strength training, you must advance.

This entails consistently increasing the intensity of your exercise by utilising larger weights. Your muscles will expand and maintain their strength as a result. Additionally, you'll have a greater sense of independence and be able to age gracefully without worrying about falling. You'll get a tremendous sense of pride and achievement from it as well.

HOW TO ADVANCE

You should begin performing each exercise with weights that you can lift at least ten times with only moderate difficulty after around the first week of strength training. If you are unable to perform a certain exercise eight times in a row, the weight you are using can be too heavy. You might have to cut back.

After two weeks of strength training, you should reconsider if the weights you are using are heavy enough.

For example, you could begin doing the overhead press with weights weighing 2 pounds. You might be able to lift the 2-pound dumbbell more than 12 times with ease by the conclusion of the second week. Make sure you are performing each workout movement correctly and that your body is in the proper position (this is referred to as having excellent form). Now you should see how the exercise feels with 3-pound weights.

If you are in good health, consistently work out, and a particular exercise feels too easy, it could be time to switch to higher weights. If you are able to complete an exercise more than ten or twelve times with the same results, it is too easy with the weights you've been utilising up until this point. If you have been ill, are injured, or your muscles are extremely sore, do not advance.

My Aunt Sarah, at the age of 65, was determined to prove that age was just a number. She began her strength training journey with scepticism but soon found herself hooked. Over the course of a year, she transformed her life. Sarah not only gained muscle and strength, but she also improved her bone density, balance, and overall well-being. Today, at 70, Sarah continues to inspire her friends with her dedication and vibrant energy. The last party we attended together, I was shocked at the way she was happy and dancing. Nobody would believe she's 70.

This real-life success story demonstrates that strength training is not just for the young; it's a pathway to a healthier, more vibrant life, regardless of age.

# Chapter 5: Staying Motivated and Consistent

Seniors can keep their independence and enjoy several health benefits from physical activity. Try to prioritise exercising. Recall that one of the most crucial things you can do every day to preserve and enhance your health is to remain active. To maintain your motivation to workouts:

1.Establish Specific, Achievable Strength Training Goals: Identify objectives that are appropriate for your age and level of fitness.

2.Make a Routine: Make a regular exercise plan that incorporates rest days and strength training.

3.Mix Up Your Workouts: To keep things fresh and avoid monotony, switch up your workouts from time to time.

4.Track Your Progress: To keep track of your progress over time, keep a workout book to record your gains.

5.Find a Workout Partner: Exercising alongside a friend can help with accountability and inspiration.

6.Put safety first: Pay attention to form, wear the right gear, and pay attention to your body to avoid injuries.

7.Reward Yourself: To show yourself appreciation for your hard work, mark your accomplishments with non-food treats.

8.Keep Up: To stay motivated and comprehend the advantages of strength training for seniors, keep up your education on the subject.

9.Adopt a Positive Attitude: Remain upbeat, exercise patience, and resist the need to let brief setbacks depress you.

10.Look for easy methods to enjoy working out.

# 5.1 Tracking Your Fitness Gains.

1.Establish Baseline Metrics: Let's begin by recording your initial strength, including how much weight you can lift and how many reps you can complete. This acts as a starting point for monitoring advancement.

2.Keep a Workout notebook: To document your training sessions, keep a workout notebook. Take note of the movements, repetitions, sets, and weight used. This facilitates monitoring your progress over time.

3.Establish Achievable and Specific Goals: Establish measurable objectives for your strength training. For instance, set a three-month goal to improve your workouts by 10%. Having specific goals inspires you to strive toward them.

4.Track Your Development Over Time: Examine your exercise log on a regular basis to determine how you're doing. Observe patterns in the rise in weight or repetitions, and acknowledge even the little successes.

5.Evaluate Functional Strength: An important aspect of strength training for seniors is their ability to function. Keep track of advancements in routine tasks like carrying groceries, ascending stairs, or lowering yourself out of a chair.

6.Seniors should pay attention to their bodies. Listen to Your Body. Keep an eye out for any pain or discomfort and modify your training accordingly. Safety should always be the top consideration.

7.Frequent Evaluations: Take into account routine evaluations conducted by a fitness specialist. They can evaluate your strength and provide advice on how to modify your routine to get better results.

8.Nutrition and Recuperation: Monitoring your progress depends greatly on your diet and recuperation. Make sure you're getting enough sleep and nutrients to promote the growth of your muscles.

9.Adapt and Change: Your fitness requirements may vary as you become older. As necessary, modify your workout regimen and keep tabs on your advancement.

10.Remain Consistent: Monitoring and attaining fitness improvements require consistency. To stay on track, follow your regimen and make adjustments as needed.

**Everything we do is much easier when we have high strength!**

**Life is a lot simpler!**

# Conclusion

It could be really tempting to strive for high goals, like lifting a specific amount of weight. However, it's actually more beneficial to ascertain your initial motivation for continuing to be strong and energetic.

Think about your goals and needs at this point in your life. Why is training necessary? The intended goal should be reflected in the strength and conditioning program.

The potential for long-term sickness is also quite important. As you age, you become more vulnerable to disease and other health issues. This may make it more difficult for you to exercise.

You should also encourage a calm, healthy mind, meditation practices like yoga and tai chi.

The ability to move functionally and go about your daily life with energy is, above all, what it means to be strong for seniors.

It's now YOUR turn to become stronger and maintain that strength even above 60.

There is a lot to process and do here, so try to keep things as easy as possible. Select an exercise regimen, be consistent, and keep moving forward. Yea! Eat healthily as well!

Your body will become stronger if you adhere to the basic strength formula. And soon long, you'll start to experience this.

You'll notice that getting about is considerably easier.

You'll begin to realise all of the advantages that come with increased muscular mass and strength.

You'll begin to appear and feel younger than you actually are!

Enjoy the process of becoming a stronger, healthier, and more fit version of yourself.

Stay joyful!

And never stop pushing yourself!

# ✦ MY WORKOUT *log*

| DAY | ACTIVITIES | TIME | REPS |
|-----|-----------|------|------|
| DAY:1 | | | |
| DAY:2 | | | |
| DAY:3 | | | |
| DAY:4 | | | |
| DAY:5 | | | |
| DAY:6 | | | |

| NOTES |
|-------|
| |

# ✦✦ MY WORKOUT *log*

| DAY | ACTIVITIES | TIME | REPS |
|---|---|---|---|
| DAY:7 | | | |
| DAY:8 | | | |
| DAY:9 | | | |
| DAY:10 | | | |
| DAY:11 | | | |
| DAY:12 | | | |

| NOTES |
|---|
| |

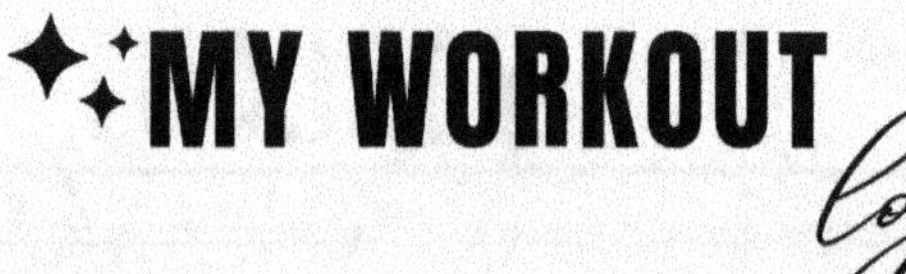


| DAY | ACTIVITIES | TIME | REPS |
| --- | --- | --- | --- |
| DAY:13 | | | |
| DAY:14 | | | |
| DAY:15 | | | |
| DAY;16 | | | |
| DAY:17 | | | |
| DAY:18 | | | |

| NOTES |
| --- |
| |

# ✦ MY WORKOUT *log*

| DAY | ACTIVITIES | TIME | REPS |
|-----|-----------|------|------|
| DAY:19 | | | |
| DAY:20 | | | |
| DAY:21 | | | |
| DAY:22 | | | |
| DAY:23 | | | |
| DAY:24 | | | |

| NOTES |
|-------|
| |

# ✦✦MY WORKOUT *log*

| DAY | ACTIVITIES | TIME | REPS |
|---|---|---|---|
| DAY:25 | | | |
| DAY:26 | | | |
| DAY:27 | | | |
| DAY:28 | | | |
| DAY:29 | | | |
| DAY:30 | | | |

| NOTES |
|---|
| |

www.ingramcontent.com/pod-product-compliance
Lightning Source LLC
Chambersburg PA
CBHW050843260726

48660CB00006B/2404